FOOD FOR THE BRAIN

DIET AND RECIPES TO KEEP YOUR BRAIN
HEALTHY AND IMPROVE MENTAL FOCUS

JOSEPH VEEBE

Books in this Series:

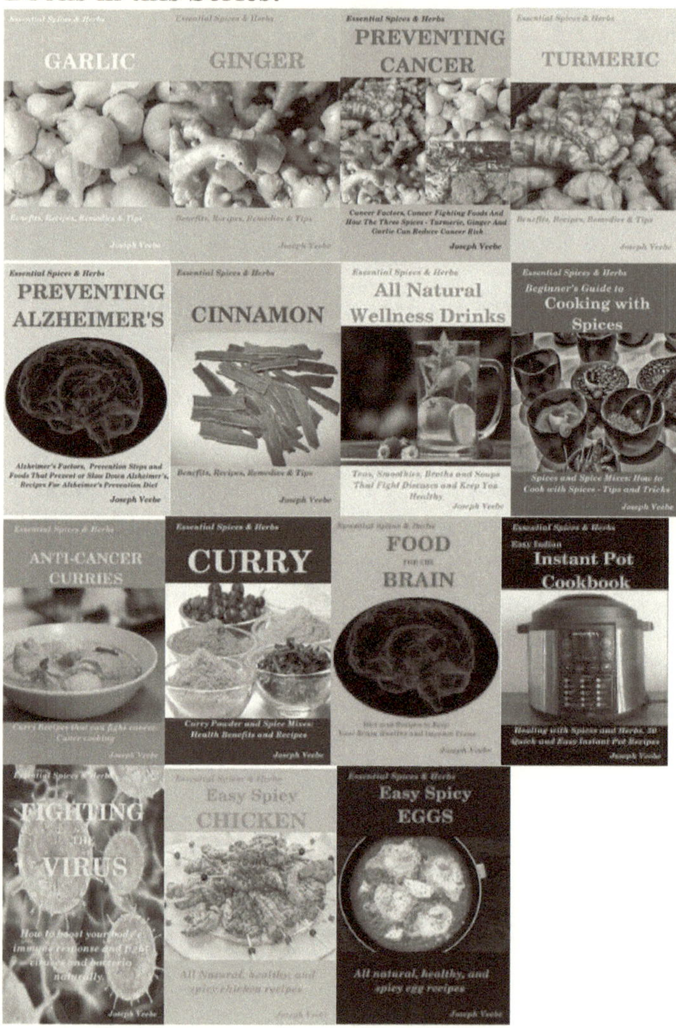

TABLE OF CONTENTS

Table of Contents...3

Chapter 1. Introduction 7

Introduction 7

Diet..9

Chapter 2. Brain Healthy Foods................................11

Anti-inflammatory properties 11

Antioxidant properties 12

Heart health 12

Immune system and infections 13

Brain Food #1: Berries..14

Brain Food #2: Nuts & Seeds....................................14

Brain Food #3: Leafy Greens....................................15

Brain Food #4: Tea..16

Brain Food #5: Coffee 17

**Brain Food #6: Healthful Unrefined Oils – Olive Oil &
Coconut Oil**...17

Brain Food #7: Dark Chocolate................................18

Brain Food #8: Avocados...18

Brain Food #9: Broccoli..19

Brain Food #10: Eggs 19

Brain Food #11: Colorful Fruits & Veggies 19

Brain Food #12: Oily Fish 20

Brain Food #13: Fermented Foods............................21

Brain Food #14: Spices 22

Brain Food #15: Herbs 25

Chapter 3. The Mediterranean Diet 28

What constitutes a Mediterranean diet? 28

4 Things to Keep in Mind 30

Mediterranean Recipe *Ideas* for the Brain 31

    Scrambled Eggs 31

    Vegetable Omelet 32

    Baked Salmon 34

    Kale Chips 35

    Oven-Baked Salmon 36

    Lamb Chops 37

    Baked Chicken Breast 38

    Chickpeas and broccoli 39

    Tuscan Tuna Salad 40

    Garlic Shrimp 41

    Baked Brussels Sprouts 41

    Mediterranean Diet – Things to Avoid 43

Chapter 4. DASH Diet 44

    What Constitutes a DASH Diet? 45

    4 Things to Keep in Mind 45

Why is DASH Diet Good for Your Brain? 46

Comparing DASH and Mediterranean Diets 47

DASH Diet Brain Food Ideas 48

    Easy Vegetable Omelet 48

    Chicken and Rice Soup 49

Healthy Chicken Salad..50

Healthy Shrimp and Asparagus Salad................................51

Roasted Salmon with Brain boosting spices and herbs 52

Chipotle Shrimp...53

Tuna stuffed Pita Pockets...54

Chapter 5. Brain-Boosting Drinks Recipe Ideas.............55

Teas..55

Basic Spice Teas..55

Teas with Natural Brain Boosting Ingredients.............56

Smoothie Ideas..57

Very Berry Smoothie...57

Beetroot and Carrot Smoothie...58

Green Smoothie with Garlic, Ginger, and Turmeric....58

Tropical Smoothie...59

Green Smoothie...60

Very Berry Smoothie...60

Avocado and Greek Yogurt Drink....................................61

Brain Healthy Broth Ideas..61

Spicy Vegan Broth..61

Bone Broths...63

Chapter 6. Brain Boosting Asian Recipe Ideas...............67

Spinach/Red Chard Stir Fry..67

Salmon with Green Mango..68

Broccoli Stir Fry..70

Coconut Curry Chicken..71

Kale and Chicken Fry 73

Chapter 7: Brain Boosting Supplements 75

Chapter 8: Summary 80

Disclaimer 83

Appendix i. Sources And References 85

Preview of Other Books in this Series 88

CHAPTER 1. INTRODUCTION

INTRODUCTION

The human body's capabilities decline as we age. Changes due to age affects all of the body's organs, cells, and tissues. Aging cells and tissues cause deterioration of the body's functions – both physical and mental.
As the cells age, they die to make way for new cells or simply die as they are programmed to do so by the body's genes. In some cases, cells die not due to age, but due to damage caused to them by harmful substances such as chemicals, radiation, sunlight, chemotherapy drugs or by free radicals produced by the cell's normal operation.

Cell death has many different implications. Loss of muscle tissues, shrinkage of the brain, reduced physical and mental capabilities are most common. Most people, with an active lifestyle, and exercise can slow down the loss of physical capabilities. However, slowing down the decline of the mind and the brain will take a lot more effort.

While it is normal to have your physical and mental abilities somewhat slow down with age, diseases such as Alzheimer's, and Parkinson's impact these declines even more.

With Alzheimer's, the rate of progressive decline in brain function is slow at the onset, but it gets worse with time and age. Brain function decline accelerates, and more and more brain cells eventually die over time.

In a normal brain (one not impacted by Alzheimer's or dementia); your brain may compensate for the loss of nerve cells in many ways:

- As the brain loses some of its nerve cells, it attempts to make connections between remaining nerve cells
- The brain may form totally new nerve cells especially, in cases, where one is learning a new language, a new musical instrument, or something that has not been done. Learning something new most often results in new brain connections and new nerve cells.
- Also, some of brain's "unused" or redundant cells come into play as they are now activated

Besides losing cells, and brain attempting to compensate them, there may be other impacts to the brain due to age such as:

- Blood flow to the brain decreases
- Nerve cells may lose some of the signal receptors for messages coming out of senses such as eyes, ear, skin, etc.
- Nerves conduct/transmit signals more slowly. This can cause a slower response, or increased reaction time or slow reflexes
- Short term memory, vocabulary, ability to learn new things are impacted

With regular exercises, strength training, practicing martial arts, and other physical activities can arrest the physical decline. This book's primary focus is on managing decline in mental and brain function through diet.

DIET

Diet has an important role to play in keeping your mind/brain and body healthy and sharp as we age. While one may not have full control of many of the environmental and genetic factors that determine their health, most have full control over our diet and what we eat or drink. A combination of diet and exercise can help prevent many diseases such as cancer, heart disease, Alzheimer's, and others. There are studies conducted that suggest the strong link between other physical disorders or diseases and the diseases of the brain. Inflammation in the brain and oxidative damage to brain cells impact brain health.

Several studies have been conducted on the relationship between diet and cognitive decline and found that eating the Mediterranean diet has significantly reduced the risk of cognitive impairment and Alzheimer's disease. Similarly, a South Asian diet that includes a lot of spices and herbs seems to help reduce the risk as well.

Studies have also shown that the DASH diet (Dietary Approaches to Stop Hypertension) has benefits for the brain. The DASH diet promotes fruits and vegetables, low-fat dairy products, whole grains, fish, nuts, and seeds.

Here are some recommendations on dieting:

- Avoid foods that cause inflammation such as sugars and refined carbs (white rice, white/bleached flour, pasta).

- Include anti-inflammatory foods (including spices and herbs) into the diet.

- Eat a lot of fish. Omega-3 fats containing DHA help prevent Alzheimer's and dementia by countering plaque formation. Include oily fishes like salmon, tuna, sardines, mackerel, trout, etc. in your diet.

- Eat a lot of fruits and vegetables, especially colorful vegetables.

- Include the Mediterranean diet as part of your diet regiment.

- Practice the DASH diet.

- Eat whole foods and grains.

- Drink more tea.

- Eat more nuts and seeds.

- Avoid fast foods, fried foods, and packaged foods.

- Avoid processed foods.

- Eat foods that strengthen your digestive system and consequently improve your immunity.

- Eat fresh meals.

- Cook at home.

CHAPTER 2. BRAIN HEALTHY FOODS

As stated before, with age, the various cells in our bodies, including within the brain, age with us. We can observe the old age in people by looking at their face and body – sagging muscles, wrinkled skin, etc. The same is true for the brain; there are shrinkages and dead cells in the brain, too. Studies have shown that by incorporating superfoods and smart foods, one can increase the chances of arresting, maintaining or even reversing the aging of both body and brain.

Below are four main characteristics of the foods that help maintain a healthy brain and provide neuroprotection.

ANTI-INFLAMMATORY PROPERTIES

Inflammation plays an important role in the natural healing process of the human body. It helps to defend against harmful invaders in our bodies such as bacteria that cause infection. Inflammation also helps the body carry out wound repair. Without inflammation, foreign invaders could cause damage to our bodies and ultimately kill us.

While short term, controlled inflammation is beneficial, it can become a major problem when it becomes chronic, such as arthritis. Chronic inflammation plays a major role in many declining brain function, neurodegenerative conditions, Alzheimer's, and other diseases. Most anti-inflammatory foods are, therefore, brain-healthy foods. By fighting inflammation that damages cells and weakens the body's immune system, these foods help improve the overall health including that of the brain.

ANTIOXIDANT PROPERTIES

Oxidative damage caused by free radicals (highly reactive molecules with unpaired electrons) contributes to the risk of cancers, heart disease, diabetes, and Alzheimer's as well as age-related macular degeneration. Free radicals tend to react with important organic substances, such as fatty acids, proteins, or DNA, causing oxidative damage.

Antioxidants help neutralize free radicals and reduce the risk of oxidative damage. They "clean up" free radicals by interacting and forming harmless substances, thereby protecting healthy cells. There are several vitamins and supplements that are known to have antioxidant properties such as vitamins C and E and beta carotene. Many of the fruits (berries, grapes, etc.) and vegetables (kale, artichokes, bell pepper, etc.) contain antioxidants. Nuts such as walnuts and beverages such as tea and coffee also contain antioxidants. Antioxidants are often added to packaged food products to keep them from interacting with air.

By incorporating foods that have antioxidant properties, one can help reduce cell damage to the body and brain.

HEART HEALTH

As several independent researches have shown, there is a strong connection between cardiovascular health and the health of the brain. Foods that help reduce cholesterol and hypertension and improve circulation and blood flow to the brain help improve brain health as well.

IMMUNE SYSTEM AND INFECTIONS

Foods that have the capability to fight infections, boost the immune system, and strengthen your gut are key in fighting many health conditions. A body that is weak in its defenses against foreign invaders is always at high risk for cancer, Alzheimer's, and many other diseases. A significant part of the body's immunity results from a healthy gut, and thus maintaining a healthy digestive system enhances the body's overall immunity and helps reduce the risk of diseases.

The next several sections describe various foods that improve brain health and prevent cognitive decline.

BRAIN FOOD #1: BERRIES

All berries are rich in antioxidants, which help neutralize free radicals in the body that usually cause cell damage. Cell damage in the brain due to oxidative stress is considered one of the reasons for cognitive decline, Alzheimer's, and dementia.

The main phytochemicals in berries are called anthocyanins. These antioxidants can counteract and neutralize free radicals. Berries are rich in other nutrients such as vitamin C, fiber, and minerals which can also fight brain cell damage.

The recommended list:

- Blueberries
- Blackberries
- Raspberries
- Strawberries
- Acai berries
- Goji berries
- Cherries

While all berries are rich in antioxidants, **blueberries** are especially good for the brain.

Suggestions:
Eat them raw. Add them to smoothies or juice them. Make sure to wash them thoroughly before eating.

BRAIN FOOD #2: NUTS & SEEDS

If you have not incorporated nuts and seeds into your diet, you should seriously consider adding them. At least 2-3 handfuls of nuts and seeds a week will provide you immense benefits.

Walnuts are especially good for brain health. Nuts have Vitamin E and also omega-3 fatty acids that help protect you from Alzheimer's by improving cognitive function and mental alertness. Some of these nuts also help prevent heart disease.

The recommended list:

- Walnuts
- Pecans
- Almonds
- Brazil nuts
- Peanuts
- Cashews
- Flax seeds
- Chia seeds
- Hemp seeds
- Sunflower seeds
- Pumpkin seeds

Suggestions:
Make it point to eat a handful of seeds/nuts every day. Walnuts are especially good for you. Replace your unhealthful snacks with nuts and seeds. Add them to smoothies. Top cereal bowls with nuts and berries. Snack on them instead of potato chips or other junk foods.

BRAIN FOOD #3: LEAFY GREENS

Dark leafy green vegetables have been getting more and more attention lately for their health benefits. Dark green leafy vegetables have a wide range of carotenoids such lutein and zeaxanthin, along with saponins and flavonoids in addition to vitamin A and K. A study conducted on the older population found that people who consumed at least one serving a day of leafy vegetables experienced slower mental decline than those who ate no vegetables.

The recommended list:

- Kale (all types – green, red, Lacinato)
- Spinach
- Chard
- Collard greens
- Mustard greens
- Seaweed (technically not a leafy green)

Suggestions:
Make them part of smoothies and salads. Sauté them with onions, garlic, ginger, etc. Add some turmeric and coconut powder. Cream them or toss some chopped greens into your meat preparations. Kale is especially good and contains 600 percent of the daily allowance of vitamins A and K in one cup.

BRAIN FOOD #4: TEA

The antioxidant chemicals (catechins) in teas have the ability to scavenge for free radicals in the body and neutralize them. Tea, with its antioxidant properties and a modest amount of caffeine, can help maintain focus and enhance memory and mood. Of all the tea varieties, **green tea** offers the most promise and according to some researchers, catechins can block amyloid plaque formation.

The recommended list:

- Green tea
- Black tea
- Chamomile tea
- Dandelion tea
- Essiac tea

Suggestions:
Make a couple of cups of tea a day as part of your daily routine. Drink freshly brewed instead of store bought (which probably is not beneficial and often contains too much sugar).

BRAIN FOOD #5: COFFEE

Coffee improves focus and helps boost memory. A Harvard study found that people who drink 3-5 cups of coffee daily have a lower risk of developing neurological diseases. Coffee contains an anti-inflammatory substance called chlorogenic acid which helps counter chronic inflammation.

BRAIN FOOD #6: HEALTHFUL UNREFINED OILS – OLIVE OIL & COCONUT OIL

Using unrefined oils such as coconut oil and extra virgin olive oil instead of refined oils can help improve the immune system. Cod liver oil (taken by the spoonful as a supplement) also has great health benefits. They all also have Omega-3 fatty acids that can help nourish the cells in your body and keep them healthy, prevent oxidation, and improve your brain function.

Olive oil is almost always used for cooking as part of Mediterranean food preparations. Coconut oil is used in cooking of some of the South Asian cuisines.

Suggestions:
Use these unrefined oils for cooking, baking, and making salad dressings.

BRAIN FOOD #7: DARK CHOCOLATE

Dark chocolate has powerful antioxidant and anti-inflammatory properties. It contains several natural brain-boosting compounds including small amounts of caffeine. Caffeine improves focus, concentration, and mood by stimulating the production of endorphins.

Suggestions:
Remember that only unprocessed or minimally processed dark chocolate (at least 70% cocoa) provides these benefits. Milk chocolates and white chocolates that you buy from the supermarket are usually heavily processed and do not provide the same benefits. An ounce of dark chocolate a day can provide immense benefits to improving brain health.

BRAIN FOOD #8: AVOCADOS

Avocados contain many essential nutrients such as vitamin B, vitamin C, vitamin K, and **folate.** In addition, avocados contain "good" fat that helps to stabilize blood sugar levels. Overall, these nutrients in avocados improve cognitive function, memory, and focus. Avocados also help prevent blood clots and protect against stroke.

Suggestions:

Include avocados in your daily salads, guacamole or as part of breakfast.

BRAIN FOOD #9: BROCCOLI

Broccoli contains high vitamin K and **choline** that will help improve memory and focus. It also contains high levels of vitamin C and fiber. It is a superfood that is great for preventing both cancer and Alzheimer's

BRAIN FOOD #10: EGGS

Eggs contain several nutrients that are important for brain health such as vitamins B6, B12, **folate,** and **choline.** All of these are very important nutrients for brain health and eggs are the easiest way to get them in your diet.

BRAIN FOOD #11: COLORFUL FRUITS & VEGGIES

One of the oft-made suggestions for healthy eating is the notion of "eating the colors of the rainbow." Brightly colored vegetables and fruits carry abundant phytochemicals that are full of carotenoid antioxidants and other essential vitamins.

Beta-carotene is one of the many carotenoids found in colored vegetables. It has been studied and found to have benefits in fighting cancers of the eye, skin, and other vital organs in the body besides being helpful in detoxification and the boosting of the immune system.

Below are some common fruits and vegetables that are colorful which should find a way into one's daily diet plans. Many of these foods have been shown to fight several cancers such as stomach, ovarian, breast, and lung cancers.

Pink/Red – Tomatoes, watermelon, red chard, pomegranate, cherries, strawberries, apples, bell peppers, raspberries, and grapefruit.

Blue/Purple – Eggplant, grapes, beets, red cabbage, purple cauliflower, blueberries, and prunes.

Yellow/Orange – Orange, apricots, papaya, mango, banana, pineapple, carrot, pumpkins, and squash.

Green – Bright green leafy vegetables - kale, spinach, peppers, celery, and artichokes.

Suggestions:
Make it a point to eat one or two servings of colored vegetables/fruits a day. Fruits may be part of smoothies; vegetables may be combined with other spices/herbs or eaten as part of a salad.

BRAIN FOOD #12: OILY FISH

The body needs essential fatty acids such as omega-3 fatty acids EPA (eicosatetraenoic acid) and DHA (docosahexaenoic acid), and oily deep-water fish are the best naturally occurring and easy to absorb source of these fatty acids. These are very important for the body's general wellbeing but especially so for the brain, heart, and joints. Some studies have linked low DHA levels to increased risk of dementia, memory loss, and Alzheimer's.

Oily fishes such as salmon, trout, mackerel, sardines, and herring are excellent sources of omega-3 essential acids. According to a study conducted by Tufts University in Boston, participants who ate at least 3 servings of oily fish a week had a 50% lower risk of Alzheimer's disease and dementia.

The fish, caught-wild, have more omega-3 and fewer toxins than farmed fish. So, buy wild-caught versions of these fish whenever possible.

While some nuts and seeds (also good brain foods) such as walnuts, flaxseeds, etc. also are rich in omega-3, they lack the EPA and DHA components in a readily available form for the body to absorb compared to the oily fishes.

Suggestions:

Consume 2-3 servings of wild-caught salmon, sardines or other oily fish every week.

BRAIN FOOD #13: FERMENTED FOODS

Fermented foods do not directly boost memory, concentration or brain health. Fermented foods are extremely helpful to maintain a healthier gut or digestive system. A healthier gut is greatly important for overall health, improved immunity, and increased ability to fight inflammation including that of the brain. This is the reason for including the group of fermented foods in this section.

There are trillions of microorganisms living in our bodies. Most of them live in our gut or digestive system. These "good bacteria" living in our gut contribute to digestion, help improves immunity and are hugely important to maintaining our health and our bodies' ability to fight disease.

Fermented foods are rich in probiotics and eating fermented food is a sure way to improve immunity and help digestion.

The recommended list:

- Yogurt – provides billions of probiotic cultures

- Kefir – fermented milk drink abundant in probiotics
- Kombucha - fermented tea
- Raw non-pasteurized cheese – provides active cultures
- Sauerkraut – made of fermented cabbage
- Kimchi – Korean version of sauerkraut; fermented vegetables including cabbage
- Pickles – pickle anything and it is good for your gut
- Miso – made of fermented soybeans with barley/brown rice and koji; a traditional Japanese dish/seasoning
- Tempeh – a fermented soybeans product; a traditional soybean product of Indonesia

Suggestions:
Include 2-3 servings of one or more of the fermented foods in your diet a week.

BRAIN FOOD #14: SPICES

Many spices have significant anti-inflammatory and antioxidant capabilities that are proven to be also neuroprotective. In this author's opinion, the top spices for neuroprotection are:

- Turmeric
- Cinnamon
- Ginger
- Garlic

Of course, there are other spices with anti-inflammatory and antioxidant properties that are good for the brain. But I consider these spices to be spices that are easy to incorporate in everyday meals.

Turmeric

Turmeric is a well-known spice in Asian cooking, especially in South Asia. Turmeric comes from the root of the turmeric plant, which is part of the ginger family. The turmeric root is cleaned, dried, and ground to create the yellow turmeric powder. Turmeric is used as an herbal supplement, added to flavor food as part of curry powder or as a standalone spice, added to cosmetics, or used as a food coloring. Turmeric is also used as a skin treatment and beauty enhancer.

The main active ingredient in turmeric is called curcumin, which has very powerful medicinal properties. However, there are two challenges in fully realizing the benefits of turmeric. First, the curcumin content is only about 3% of turmeric by weight. Second, curcumin is not easily absorbed by the body. Curcumin absorption can be substantially enhanced by consuming black pepper, which contains *piperine*, along with turmeric. Also, fatty foods have proven to aid curcumin absorption as well. To consume a sufficient dosage of curcumin, a combination of curcumin/turmeric extract supplements along with a diet prepared with turmeric is recommended.

Turmeric is a rich source of many essential vitamins and minerals; it does not contain any cholesterol but is an excellent source of antioxidants and dietary fiber, which helps to control bad cholesterol levels.

Turmeric's antioxidant levels are one of the highest among popular spices and herbs and is an excellent brain-boosting substance on many levels.

Ginger

Ginger (*Zingiber officinale*) is a flowering plant whose root is widely used as a spice and traditional medicine over thousands of years in Asia. Ginger belongs to the same family as turmeric and cardamom.

Ginger is widely used in Asian cooking, especially in China and India. While turmeric, which belongs to the same family as ginger, is mostly used in the powder form, ginger is used as a fresh ingredient in most cooking.

The main bioactive active ingredient in ginger is called gingerol and it has very powerful medicinal properties, including antioxidant and anti-inflammatory properties. Ginger is used in several alternative/traditional medicines in the East.

Garlic

Garlic is part of the *Allium* (onion) family and is closely related to shallots, onions, Chinese onions, chives, and leeks. The main active ingredient in garlic is called polysulphide allicin and is responsible primarily for its medicinal properties. This compound, allicin, formed when garlic cloves are chopped or crushed, not only provides the medicinal properties but the distinct taste and smell as well.

Cinnamon

Cinnamon is not only nutrient-rich but also has many health benefits. Cinnamon is used in Ayurveda as a remedy for toothache, respiratory tract infections, chest congestion, stomach ailments, and cold and flu. Cinnamon has antibacterial, anti-viral, and antifungal properties.

Many of the recent studies have found several additional health benefits such as antioxidant, anti-inflammatory, and anticoagulant properties, as well as reducing cholesterol and blood sugar levels. Other studies have found benefits such as slowing down cognitive decline, HIV treatment, and anti-cancer properties.

Cinnamon is known to have one of the highest antioxidant rates among the many commonly used foods. In a study of 26 common spices and herbs on their antioxidant properties, cinnamon came out on top eclipsing garlic, oregano, thyme, and cloves.

Compounds in cinnamon are being studied for their ability to stop the buildup of tau proteins that cause tangles in the brain, which are considered a precursor to Alzheimer's.

BRAIN FOOD #15: HERBS

Like spices, many herbs also have neuroprotective properties. The most significant among them are:

- Rosemary
- Sage
- Ginkgo Biloba
- Lion's Mane
- Bacopa Monnieri or Brahmi
- Ashwagandha
- Ginseng
- Gotu Kola or Indian Pennywort
- Lemon balm

Rosemary has neurogenerative properties like many other herbs. The main ingredient in rosemary, called carnosic acid, neutralizes free radicals in the brain and helps improve brain health, fight against strokes, fight Alzheimer's and arrest the aging of the brain.

Sage is considered to possess memory-enhancing properties and likely to be beneficial for Alzheimer's patients based on evidence-based studies. Rosemary and sage may be added to roasted chicken, tomato sauce, and soups.

Ginkgo biloba is commonly used as a treatment for dementia in Chinese traditional medicine. Ginkgo Biloba may improve cognitive function by stimulating blood flow to the brain.

Lion's Mane is a white shaggy mushroom that resembles a lion's mane. Lion's Mane is used in ancient Chinese medicine and may improve cognitive function, prevent memory loss, and reduce symptoms of depression and anxiety, among other benefits.

Bacopa Monnieri or Brahmi is used in traditional Ayurvedic medicine for its cognition and memory-enhancing properties. A 2001 study found that Brahmi significantly improved learning and memory retention over placebo.

Ashwagandha is an ayurvedic herb that may help the aging brain in a couple of ways – 1) inhibit the formation of beta-amyloid plaques and 2) prevent oxidative damage to brain cells. Ashwagandha is also helpful in relaxation and anxiety relief.

Ginseng, one of the most popular herbs in Chinese medicine, contains anti-inflammatory compounds called ginsenosides which have shown to reduce the beta-amyloid build up in the brain.

The best way to consume ginkgo biloba, lion's mane, ashwagandha, and ginseng are through extracts and supplements. Extracts, supplements, and tea formulations of these ancient herbs are available in many online stores including Amazon.

Gotu Kola is used in both Chinese traditional medicine and Ayurveda to improve mental clarity. Some animal studies have shown that this herb may also help fight oxidative damage to brain cells. Gotu Kola is helpful in maintaining nervous system health.

Lemon balm is often taking in tea form can help reduce anxiety and improve sleep function. Lemon balm may help improve cognition.

CHAPTER 3. THE MEDITERRANEAN DIET

The awareness about the benefits of the Mediterranean diet originated as a result of the Seven Country Study conducted in the 1970s. It was found that the diet consumed throughout the Mediterranean region had a beneficial effect on overall health and especially on heart health. The reason to the cover Mediterranean diet as part of brain food is simply that this diet is widely considered as one of the healthiest diets by experts in the diet and nutrition field. Mediterranean diet is considered as an anti-aging, brain-boosting, and overall healthy diet for mind and body. This type of diet includes vegetables, legumes, fruits, nuts, beans, fish, and whole grains. The diet is cooked or consumed with good fats such as olive oil.

Mediterranean diet is usually free from bad cholesterols, is antioxidant-rich, and include anti-inflammatory foods. By following this diet, one can reduce the risk of cardiovascular diseases, Alzheimer's and Parkinson's and possibly prolong your life and improve quality of life.

WHAT CONSTITUTES A MEDITERRANEAN DIET?

As stated above Mediterranean diet usually consists of the following:
1. Fruits
   - Berries
   - Figs
   - Dates
   - Plums
   - Oranges
   - Peaches
   - Grapes

- Bananas
- Apples
- Apricot
- Melons
- Avocados

2. Vegetables
   - Artichokes
   - Olives
   - Broccoli, Cabbage, Green Beans
   - Eggplant
   - Onions, leaks, Garlic
   - Beets, Carrots, Peas, Squash
   - Leafy Greens
   - Tomato, Bell peppers, Mushrooms
   - Yams, Sweet Potatoes

3. Nuts and Seeds
   - Almonds, Cashews, Walnuts, Peanuts
   - Pumpkin seeds, Sunflower seeds, Flax seeds

4. Grains
   - Brown or Wild Rice
   - Quinoa
   - Barley
   - Couscous
   - Oatmeal
   - Whole-grain breads
   - Pasta

5. Beans
   - Black beans, Chickpeas,
   - Pinto beans, white beans, Lentils

6. Dairy
   - Eggs

- Plain Greek Yogurt
- Cheese
- Whole Milk

7. Oils
    - Extra virgin olive oil
    - Avocado oil
    - Grape seed oil

8. Meat and Fish
    - Oily fish such as Salmon, Mackerel, sardines,
    - Shrimp, Scallops, Crab
    - Cod, Tuna, Tilapia
    - Chicken
    - Turkey
    - Grass-fed beef

9. Spices and Herbs
    - Basil, Cilantro, Parsley, Rosemary
    - Sage, Thyme, Oregano, Mint, Bay leaves
    - Chilies, Black pepper, Cumin

4 THINGS TO KEEP IN MIND

1. Eat nuts, fruits, and vegetables every day
2. Eat fish at least 2-3 times a week. Substitute red meat and poultry with seafood
3. Eat dairy & poultry in moderation, red meat rarely
4. Cook with good oils such olive or avocado and avoid butter, ghee, margarine

MEDITERRANEAN RECIPE *IDEAS* FOR THE BRAIN

The recipes listed below are essentially a result of applying Mediterranean diet principles in cooking with brain-healthy ingredients. The recipes are presented here are for you to try from a "Food for the Brain" perspective than an authentic range of Mediterranean recipes.

SCRAMBLED EGGS

Ingredients:
- 1 tablespoon olive oil
- 1 bunch spring onions chopped
- ¼ cup green olives chopped
- 1 tomato chopped
- 3 eggs
- ¼ tsp black pepper powder
- Salt to taste
- ¼ cup Goat cheese or feta cheese (optional)

Method
1. Heat oil in a pan
2. Add chopped green onions, olives and tomatoes and saute for about 2-3 minutes
3. Stir in eggs. Mix to scramble
4. Keep stirring on medium heat until eggs cooked and scrambled well.
5. Add optional cheese and mix well
6. Sprinkle salt and pepper
7. Serve warm

Recipe Notes:

1. Vegetables may be mixed & matched to create. 2-3 combination of following chopped up vegetable may be used
   a. Baby spinach, kale, mushrooms, broccoli, cauliflower, Italian squash, onions, tomatoes, olives, artichokes, bell pepper
2. One or more of the following herbs can be added as well
   a. Cilantro, parsley, basil, mint
3. If you feel adventurous chop up and add one or more of the following
   a. Jalapeno's, ginger, garlic & turmeric powder. If turmeric powder is used, make sure to sauté it well in oil so the raw taste is removed.

VEGETABLE OMELET

Ingredients:
- 2 tablespoon olive oil
- 1 small onion chopped
- 1 clove of garlic chopped
- ¼ cup green olives chopped (canned may be used)
- ¼ cup chopped up artichoke hearts (canned may be used)
- 1 tomato chopped
- 4 eggs
- ¼ tsp black pepper powder
- Salt to taste
- 1 tablespoon shredded cheese (optional)

Method
1. Heat 1 tablespoon oil in a pan

2. Add chopped onions, olives, artichokes and tomatoes and saute for about 4-5 minutes or until vegetables are tender
3. Sprinkle salt and pepper and remove the vegetables from the pan
4. Add 1 tablespoon olive oil.
5. Beat the egg and pour into the pan. Cook for 1-2 minutes or until the edges become firm the egg begins to set.
6. Use a spatula to lift the egg from sides to make sure it is not sticking to the pan
7. Spread optional cheese and now use a spoon to place the cooked vegetable in the center of the omelet.
8. Gently fold the omelet over the vegetables. Press gently with the spatula so the vegetables are properly sandwiched between. Cook for 1-2 minutes. Turn over if needed.
9. Cut it into two halves and serve

Recipe Notes:
1. As in the previous recipe, vegetables may be mixed & matched to create. 2-3 combination of following chopped up vegetable may be used
   a. Baby spinach, kale, mushrooms, broccoli, cauliflower, zucchini, onions, tomatoes, olives, and artichokes
2. One or more of the following herbs can be added as well
   a. Cilantro, parsley, basil, mint
3. If you feel adventurous chop up and add one or more of the following

a. Jalapeno's, ginger, garlic & turmeric powder. If turmeric powder is used, make sure to saute it well in oil so the raw taste is removed.
4. Add your favorite cheese
a. Feta cheese, goat cheese, grated cheese mix

Mixing and matching the vegetables, spices & herbs and cheese, you can make many different omelets. Use your creativity and try different combinations!

BAKED SALMON

Ingredients:
- 2 tablespoon olive oil
- 1 spring onion chopped
- 1 clove of garlic chopped
- ¼ cup green olives chopped (canned may be used)
- 1 tomato chopped
- 6 oz salmon filets – 2
- ¼ tsp black pepper powder
- Salt to taste
- 1 tablespoon cilantro or basil finely chopped

Method
1. Mix all the vegetables, herbs, pepper and salt and oil
2. On an aluminum foil and put one filet on a bed of ½ of vegetable and herb mix. Spread the remaining half on top of the fish filet.
3. Fold the aluminum foil and seal the contents.
4. Bake in the oven at 450 degrees (F) for about 15 minutes

5. Let it cool for about 5-10 minutes before serving with rice.

Recipe Notes:
1. The same recipe may be used for other types of fish such as tilapia, swordfish, and tuna.
2. Other herbs such as rosemary, mint, parsley may be used.
3. Tomato may be substituted with the juice of one lime for the acid in the preparation.
4. Spices may be used. See recipes in the Indian section
5. Instead of aluminum foil, banana leaf or any other leaf may be used. In this case, use a cooking string or bakers twine to seal the contents before baking
6. This recipe takes only about 15-20 minutes, but if you want to make it even quicker. Just use some medium (or hot depending taste) salsa and black pepper mixed with olive oil on the fish and bake instead of all the other ingredients.

KALE CHIPS

Ingredients
- 1 bunch of red, green or Lacinato kale
- 2 tsp olive oil or garlic oil

Optional Ingredients
- A pinch of salt

Method

1. Preheat the oven to 350 degrees Fahrenheit (175 C.)

2. Use a knife to remove the thick stems from the leaves (the thick stems may be reused in soups or chili instead of discarding) and tear the leaves into small chip-sized pieces.
3. Put all the pieces in a mixing bowl, sprinkle with oil (olive or garlic oil), and salt (kale is a bit salty by itself so you can skip the salt depending on your taste) and mix well. Set it aside for 5 minutes before baking.
4. Bake for 10 minutes or until the kale pieces are crisp (be careful not to burn the chips).

OVEN-BAKED SALMON

Ingredients

- 4 salmon fillets (5-6 ounces each)
- 2 teaspoons olive oil
- 1 teaspoon turmeric powder
- ½ -1 teaspoon black pepper powder
- ¼ cup chopped cilantro
- ¼ parsley flakes
- 2 garlic cloves, finely chopped
- 2 teaspoons lemon juice
- ½ -1 teaspoon salt (or to taste)

Optional Ingredients

- ½ inch ginger root, grated

Method

1. Place the salmon fillets skin down on a well-greased (olive oil or butter) glass baking dish (sufficiently large to hold the 4 pieces).

2. Put the other ingredients – garlic, ginger, turmeric, black pepper, lemon juice, salt, and olive oil – in a small bowl and mix well.
3. Coat the spice, oil, and lemon mixture on each of the fillets.
4. Now cover the fillets with cilantro and parsley by sprinkling the herbs on top.
5. Bake for 18-20 minutes at 375 degrees Fahrenheit.

LAMB CHOPS

Ingredients
- 2 lb lamb chops (8-10 pieces)
- 2 tablespoons olive oil
- ½ teaspoon turmeric powder
- ½ teaspoon coriander powder
- ½ teaspoon cumin powder
- ¼ teaspoon cinnamon powder
- ½ teaspoon black pepper powder
- ½ teaspoon dried rosemary
- ¼ teaspoon dried thyme
- 2 garlic cloves, finely chopped
- 2 teaspoons lemon juice
- ½ -1 teaspoon salt (or to taste)

Optional Ingredients
- ½ inch ginger root, grated

Method
1. Combine all ingredients (except lamb) in a large enough dish. Mix well

2. Now add the lamb chops, rub all the ingredients well onto both sides. Let it sit for 4 hours or let it sit overnight.
3. Pre-heat the grill, grill for 4-5 minutes per side until both sides are nicely browned. Once the center of the chops reads 145 degrees (F), the chops are ready.

BAKED CHICKEN BREAST

Ingredients
- 4 pieces of chicken breast
- 2 tablespoons olive oil
- ½ teaspoon black pepper powder
- ½ teaspoon dried thyme
- ½ teaspoon dried oregano
- 2 garlic cloves, finely chopped
- 2 teaspoons lemon juice
- ½ -1 teaspoon salt (or to taste)

Method
1. Rub salt and pepper to both sides of the chicken breast.
2. Combine rest ingredients (except chicken) in a large enough baking dish. Mix well
3. Now add the chicken breast, rub all the ingredients well onto both sides. Let it sit for 15 minutes
4. Preheat the oven at 400 degrees(F) and bake for 30-40 minutes or until chicken is done.

CHICKPEAS AND BROCCOLI

This is an easy recipe. Several variations of the recipe is given in the recipe notes.

Ingredients
- 2 cans of chickpeas/garbanzo beans
- ¾ lb broccoli florets finely chopped
- ½ medium onion
- ½ teaspoon cumin
- ½ teaspoon dried oregano
- 2 garlic cloves, finely chopped
- 2 tablespoon olive oil
- ½ -1 teaspoon salt (or to taste)

Optional Ingredients
- ½ teaspoon turmeric
- 1 jalapeno sliced (seed out or in depending heat tolerance level)

Method
1. Heat oil in a pan and crackle cumin seeds
2. Add onion and sauté. Add optional ingredients and mix well.
3. Now add the finely chopped broccoli. Mix well.
4. Cover and cook for 3-4 minutes or until broccoli is tender to your taste
5. Add drained chickpeas. Mix well. Sprinkle oregano. Cover and cook for another 2-3 minutes

Recipe Notes:
1. The same recipe may be used for combining chickpeas with other kinds of vegetables such as:
   a. Chopped up spinach
   b. Chopped up kale

c. Chopped up zucchini
d. Chopped cauliflower
e. Chopped up bell peppers
f. Chopped mushrooms
g. Chopped up tomatoes
h. Spring onions

2. Herbs such as rosemary, mint, parsley, cilantro may be used instead of oregano or in addition to oregano
3. Spices may be used. See recipes in the Indian section. If spices such as coriander, chili, turmeric or cumin are used, make sure to fry them in olive oil along with onions to make sure spices do not taste raw.
4. Instead of vegetables, any of the following fish/meat may be used in the recipe as well:
    a. Canned tuna
    b. Canned sardines
    c. Ground chicken, turkey, of beef

If uncooked ground meat is used, make sure to cook it well before adding chickpeas

TUSCAN TUNA SALAD

Ingredients
- 3-4 cups of spinach or your favorite greens
- 1 can of (12-15 oz) white beans drained
- 1 can of white tuna in water, drained
- ½ cup cherry tomatoes halved
- 1 medium onion sliced
- 2 tablespoon olive oil (extra virgin)
- ½ teaspoon salt (or to taste)
- ¼ cup crumbled feta cheese

- 1 teaspoon lemon juice

Method
1. In a large bowl, combine all ingredients except olive oil, salt, and lemon juice and mix well.
2. Sprinkle olive oil, lemon juice and salt to taste and mix well.

GARLIC SHRIMP

Ingredients
- 1 lb. cooked shrimp
- ½ cup chopped tomatoes
- 2-3 tablespoons minced garlic
- ¼ cup chopped parsley
- 2 tablespoon olive oil (extra virgin)
- ½ teaspoon salt (or to taste)
- 1 teaspoon lemon juice

Method
1. Heat oil in a medium sized pan
2. Sauté garlic, add tomatoes mix well.
3. Add shrimp and mix well. Cook for 1-2 minutes.
4. Sprinkle parsley, lemon juice, and salt. Mix and serve

BAKED BRUSSELS SPROUTS

Ingredients

- 1-1/2 lb. Brussels sprouts washed and cut into halves
- 1-2 teaspoons minced garlic (optional)
- 3 tablespoon olive oil (extra virgin)
- ½ teaspoon salt (or to taste)
- 1 teaspoon turmeric powder
- ½ teaspoon ground black pepper
- 1 teaspoon lemon juice (optional)
- Chopped cilantro (optional)

Method

1. In a large enough bowl, toss brussels sprouts with olive oil. Make sure brussels sprouts is coated well with olive oil.
2. Sprinkle turmeric, black pepper powder, and salt. Toss again so the brussels sprouts are now coated with spices and salt.
3. Spread them evenly on a baking pan and roast/bake them for about 25-30 minutes in the oven pre-heated at 400 degrees.
4. Sprinkle optional cilantro and lemon juice and serve hot.

Recipe Notes:

1. Instead of spices, you can use a mixture of grated parmesan and breadcrumbs to coat the brussels sprouts. This will make crispy non-spicy roasted brussels sprouts.
2. Instead of fresh garlic, garlic powder may be used
3. You may try sprinkling ½ teaspoon of cumin powder before roasting

4. To make sure brussels sprouts come out crispy, make sure they evenly spread, and the pieces do not touch each other.

MEDITERRANEAN DIET – THINGS TO AVOID

1. Refined oils such as canola oil, soybean oil
2. Butter, Margarine
3. Fried foods of any kind
4. Processed meats such as hot dogs, sausages, etc.
5. Sugars – ice cream, sodas or other sugary products
6. Processed foods that contain too much sugar
7. Refined grains

CHAPTER 4. DASH DIET

Dietary Approach to Stop Hypertension on DASH is more than a diet and is essentially a lifestyle approach. DASH diet originated from a research study in the nineties on stopping or preventing hypertension by the National Heart, Lung, and Blood Institute (NHLBI). Much like the Mediterranean diet, the focus is on lifestyle changes and healthy eating including watching and controlling sodium intake which can directly cause hypertension.

According to the US Center for Disease Control, one in three adults (close to 80 million) in the US has hypertension. Hypertension can lead to the weakening of arteries resulting in higher chances of heart disease and stroke. The overall goal of a DASH diet plan is to avoid unhealthy fats, cholesterol-rich, and high sodium foods. In other words, the DASH diet focus on fresh fruits and vegetables, low-fat dairy products, lean protein, and fiber-rich foods.

As with many other diet plans, the DASH diet is about healthy, disciplined and responsible eating. Cutting fat and sodium, especially sodium from processed foods is central to DASH diet.

The DASH diet program is included in this book about brain food is simple. Research has shown that there is a strong heart to head connection. Keeping heart healthy and reducing hypertension has a direct connection to keeping the brain healthy and maintaining a sharper mind. Some studies have shown that a combination of the DASH diet and exercise resulted in improvements in executive function than just the DASH diet alone.

WHAT CONSTITUTES A DASH DIET?

As stated above DASH diet consists of a diet plan that is rich in fruits and vegetables, high fiber foods, low-fat dairy, lean protein, and very low sodium.

A recommended DASH diet broadly consists of a daily allowance of:

- 4-5 servings of vegetables (2-3 cups)
- 4-5 servings of fruits   (2-3 small fruits)
- 6-7 servings of whole grain (1/2 cup rice/pasta or noodles is one serving as is one slice of bread)
- 1-2 servings of low-fat dairy (1 cup yogurt, 1 glass milt)
- 1-2 servings lean meat or fish (3-6 ounces)
- 2-3 tablespoons of fat/oils (these include butter, margarine, mayonnaise, salad dressing, vegetable oil)
- 1 serving of nuts, seeds or beans (1/2 cup)
- 2 teaspoon or less sugar
- Less than 2000 mg of salt

Note:
This is a typical diet and depending on your weight, age, lifestyle activity, you may decrease or increase these by 25%. Consult a dietician or doctor for definite recommendations.

4 THINGS TO KEEP IN MIND

1. The first thing to keep in mind is that the DASH diet focuses on low sodium. This really means most processed products are out. Even the processed food that explicitly says low sodium probably contains more sodium than DASH diet recommendation.

2. By just practicing the low sodium diet alone can provide immense benefits since it removes a large portion of processed foods!!

3. DASH diet limits fat intake. This means low-fat dairy products and lean meat are part of DASH diet. Low-fat dairy and lean meat help overall weight loss, improve cholesterol and cardiovascular health. Improved cardiovascular health is key to improved brain health.

4. Similar to the Mediterranean diet, vegetables, fruits, and nuts are integral to the DASH diet. In fact, a majority of the daily food servings under DASH diet will fall into fruits and vegetables along with whole grains and a limited amount of meat & fish.

WHY IS DASH DIET GOOD FOR YOUR BRAIN?

While there are overall health benefits with the DASH diet, it is primarily focused on reducing hypertension and thus improving heart health. Improving heart health is vitally important for brain health. DASH diet promotes a reduction of inflammation, neutralizes free radicals due to antioxidant-rich foods, and promote weight loss. Research has shown inflammation as the major cause of a decrease in brain function. A properly maintained DASH diet helps in:

- Improving blood flow into the brain

- Reducing inflammation
- Neutralizing free radicals
- Effective in reducing the chances of plaque formation in the brain which results in cognitive decline.

While the DASH diet helps overall health, a study found that DASH diet with aerobic exercise improved cognitive function compared to a group that followed DASH alone or non-DASH diet.

COMPARING DASH AND MEDITERRANEAN DIETS

I have included both the Mediterranean and DASH diet as brain-healthy diets. If you were to compare them side by side, they are both more similar in objectives and practice than different. Both emphasis whole grains, fruits, and vegetables, both recommend avoiding red or processed meats (and other processed foods). The difference primarily is in the amount of fish and lean meat as the Mediterranean diet encourages more fish and seafood. Mediterranean diet also recommends the use of olive oil in all meal preparations and daily servings of nuts. DASH diet has a strict recommendation on sodium, usually less than 1500 mg a day for at-risk (hypertension) adults compared to the 2300 mg allowance by USDA. However, both diet plans achieve the following:

- Reduces hypertension (DASH is focused on this)
- Improves potential for weight loss
- Reduces cardiovascular risk
- Reduces chances of stroke

- Reduces chances of kidney disease
- Reduces chances of cancer, heart disease, diabetes
- Reduces inflammation
- Improves brain function

DASH DIET BRAIN FOOD IDEAS.

The recipe ideas below incorporate DASH diet principles to cooking food using ingredients known to benefit brain function and cognition (Chapter 2). As indicated under Mediterranean diet, while these recipes can be followed as is to make some delicious food, these are more of recipe ideas and reader can apply DASH diet principles to mix and match brain healthy ingredients to create additional recipes and dishes and a build a diet plan that works for them.

EASY VEGETABLE OMELET

Ingredients:
- 1 tablespoon butter
- 1 small onion chopped
- 1 clove of garlic chopped
- 1 cup baby spinach chopped
- 4 eggs
- ¼ tsp black pepper powder
- ¼ tsp cayenne pepper
- Salt to taste
- 1 tablespoon shredded cheese (optional)

Method
1. Heat butter in a pan

2. Add chopped onions, and tomatoes, cayenne pepper, black pepper powder, salt, chopped up spinach and eggs and whisk well.
3. Pour the mixture into the pan and cook on low to medium heat for 1-2 minutes or until the edges become firm the egg begins to set.
4. Use a spatula to lift the egg from sides to make sure it is not sticking to the pan
5. Switch off the heat, spread optional cheese, cover and let it sit for 1 minute for the cheese to melt
6. Cut it into two halves and serve

CHICKEN AND RICE SOUP

This is a simple and wholesome recipe that takes 15-30 minutes to prepare depending on white rice or brown rice is used.

Ingredients
- ½ cup brown rice pre-soaked
- 1 onion chopped
- 2-3 garlic cloves chopped
- ½ inch ginger grated
- 1 cup vegetables of your choice (peas, carrots, cauliflower, beans) chopped up
- 6 oz chicken breast sliced into small pieces
- 3-4 cups of clear bone broth, vegetable/chicken broth – low sodium
- 1-2 medium tomatoes sliced
- 1 tablespoon oil

Method

1. Heat oil in a saucepan, add onions, garlic, and ginger and sauté for 1-2 minutes

2. Add all the rest of the ingredients and the broth.
3. Bring to boil, cover, and cook until rice and chicken are well cooked.
4. Add salt, if you must.

Recipe Notes:

1. While brown rice is healthier, using white rice will cut down the cooking time by half
2. If an instant pot is used to cook, first sauté onions in sauté setting and then cook on high pressure for 15 minutes (brown rice) and 5 minutes (white rice)
3. Adding one chopped jalapeno provides additional heat if you like a hot version of this soup
4. Instead of tomato, you may add 1 cup of medium salsa
5. While sautéing onions, you may also add spices of your choice (turmeric, cayenne, cumin, or any other).

HEALTHY CHICKEN SALAD

Ingredients
- 4 cups of dark green leafy vegetable of your choice chopped
- ½ onion sliced
- 10-12 cherry tomatoes halved
- 1 cup cucumber
- 1 avocado, peeled, pitted and sliced
- 6 oz chicken breast sliced into small pieces
- ¼ tsp turmeric
- ¼ tsp cayenne pepper
- 2 tablespoons low-fat yogurt or 1 lemon juice
- 1 tablespoon olive oil
- Salad dressing of your choice – 1-2 tablespoon

Method

1. Mix yogurt, turmeric, cayenne pepper, and a pinch of salt to make a marinade. You can substitute yogurt with lemon juice.
2. Marinate the chicken pieces for at least 10 minutes.
3. Bake chicken on 400 degrees for 15 minutes or air fry for 10 minutes
4. Now toss all the other salad ingredients in a bowl, mix well. Add baked/air fried chicken
5. Pour dressing of your choice or enjoy as is

HEALTHY SHRIMP AND ASPARAGUS SALAD

Ingredients
- ½ lb. Asparagus spears trimmed (about 15 spears)
- ½ lb. peeled, cooked shrimp
- 10-12 cherry tomatoes halved
- 1 avocado, peeled, pitted and sliced
- 2 cup baby spinach or tender kale
- ¼ cup vinaigrette dressing of your choice
- Salt and pepper to taste

Method

1. First blanch asparagus. Boil water in a pan, add asparagus and cook for 2-3 minutes. Take them out and wash them in cold/ice water. Cut it into 1 ½ inch pieces
2. Add rest of the ingredients – shrimp, spinach/kale, tomatoes, avocados, and green onions.
3. Add dressing, salt, and pepper and toss it all together and enjoy

ROASTED SALMON WITH BRAIN BOOSTING SPICES AND HERBS

Ingredients
- 4 wild-caught salmon fillets (5-6 ounces each)
- 2 teaspoons olive oil
- ½ teaspoon turmeric powder
- ½ -1 teaspoon black pepper powder
- 2 garlic cloves, finely chopped
- 2 teaspoons lemon juice
- ½ inch ginger root, grated
- 2 springs of rosemary
- Salt to taste

Method
1. Sprinkle turmeric and pepper powder on both sides of the salmon evenly
2. Place the salmon fillets a well-greased (using 1 teaspoon olive oil) glass baking dish (sufficiently large to hold the 4 pieces).
3. Put the other ingredients – garlic, ginger, lemon juice, salt, and rest of the olive oil – in a small bowl and mix well.
4. Coat the spice, oil, and lemon mixture on each of the fillets.
5. Now cover the fillets rosemary
6. Bake for 20-22 minutes at 400 degrees Fahrenheit.

CHIPOTLE SHRIMP

Ingredients
- 1 lb raw shrimp washed, peeled and deveined, tail on
- 2 teaspoons olive oil
- ½ teaspoon turmeric powder
- ½ -1 teaspoon black pepper powder
- 1 tsp ginger-garlic paste
- 2 teaspoons lemon juice
- ½ -1 teaspoon chipotle chili powder
- Salt to taste

Method
1. Combine all ingredients except shrimp in a bowl to make a marinade. Add 1 tablespoon water if the marinade is too thick
2. Apply marinade on the shrimp and mix well so the marinade is well coated.
3. Refrigerate for 30 minutes to one hour (you can keep it overnight as well)
4. Thread the shrimp on skewers and grill until cooked

Recipe Notes:
1. You can also bake or broil the marinated shrimp in a conventional oven
2. You can also air fry the shrimp. If air frying, no need to use skewers.
3. If you want some vegetables along with shrimp, mix in cut bell peppers, zucchini, and onions along with shrimp. Thread vegetables and shrimp alternatively on the skewer and grill or bake.

TUNA STUFFED PITA POCKETS

Ingredients
- 1 cup baby spinach/ tender kale/romaine lettuce shredded
- 1 teaspoon olive oil
- ½ cup diced tomatoes
- ½ cup finely chopped bell pepper (red or yellow)
- ½ cup broccoli finely chopped
- ¼ cup onion chopped
- 12 oz low sodium while tuna in water, drained
- ¼ cup cilantro
- ¼- ½ cup low fat ranch dressing or dressing of your choice
- 3 whole-wheat pita pockets, cut into half

Method
1. Mix all ingredients together in a large bowl.
2. Stuff pita pockets with tuna salad and serve

CHAPTER 5. BRAIN-BOOSTING DRINKS RECIPE IDEAS

TEAS

As mentioned earlier, traditional teas (black, green, or white) contain antioxidants that help remove free radicals in your body and brain. The moderate amounts of caffeine in teas also help with focus and memory. The next section contains several tea ideas both traditional and others:

1. Combine traditional tea with helpful spices and herbs
2. Make teas out of natural substances that are known to help improve brain health, memory, and cognition.

BASIC SPICE TEAS

Turmeric Tea:

1. Put the ½ -1 teaspoon turmeric and ¼ teaspoon ground pepper in a cup or pot, add one spoon of water, mix and make it into a paste.
2. Boil 1-2 cups of water and add to the turmeric paste. Mix it well.
3. Strain out the turmeric pieces, if any.
4. Let it cool for a couple of minutes and add honey or brown sugar to your taste. Enjoy warm.

Ginger Tea:
1. Add 1 teaspoon grated ginger to water and boil it for a couple of minutes.
2. Let it cool down

3. Filter ginger out; add honey and lemon juice; stir and enjoy lukewarm.

Black Tea with Ginger and Cardamom:

1. Add 1 teaspoon grated ginger 2 pods of crushed cardamom to 1-2 cups of water and boil.
2. Add a black or green tea bag.
3. Let it cool for a couple of minutes.
4. Remove tea bag, filter ginger slices; add honey brown sugar to taste. Enjoy warm.

Note: Try adding 1 teaspoon lemon juice and make it part of the recipe ingredients if you like it.

TEAS WITH NATURAL BRAIN BOOSTING INGREDIENTS

The following section provides ideas of making tea out of some of the herbs and other natural substances that are known to improve brain health. As described earlier, these ingredients have high antioxidant properties and are packed with important polyphenols and phytonutrients. Some ideas for these include:

Rosemary Tea: Boil 1-2 cups of water, immerse rosemary tea bag and cover, and let it steep for 5-6 minutes. Enjoy warm.

Sage Tea: Boil 1-2 cups of water, immerse one organic sage tea bag. Cover and steep it between 3-10 minutes depending on how strong you like the tea to be. If you boil or steep it for long, the color of the tea may be become darker from yellowish and taste a little bitter.

Ginseng Tea: Boil 1-2 cups of water, immerse ginseng tea bag and cover and let it steep for 5-6 minutes. Enjoy warm.

Other Herbal Teas: Chamomile tea, dandelion tea, echinacea tea, lemon balm tea, and hibiscus tea. These teas are available to buy in many health food stores and are made similar to the recipes above.

SMOOTHIE IDEAS

The smoothie recipe ideas given below may be further enhanced by adding brain boosting supplements (please see Chapter 8) that are available in powder forms such as lions mane, ashwagandha, Gotu kola, ginseng, ginkgo biloba, turmeric, ginger or any of the other supplements described in this book. These powders may be added to smoothies to convert an ordinary smoothie to a brain-boosting one.

VERY BERRY SMOOTHIE

Berries are superfoods with many benefits including fighting cancer, anti-aging by keeping your brain young.

Ingredients
- ½ cup blueberries
- ½ cup blackberries
- ½ cup raspberries
- ½ cup strawberries
- 1 cup 2% milk or low-fat yogurt
- ½ cup ice

Method

Process all the ingredients in a blender until smooth.

BEETROOT AND CARROT SMOOTHIE

This smoothie is a potent anti-oxidant and anti-inflammatory drink. It contains vitamin A, C, and E, and iron and calcium. An excellent drink when you are down with cold, flu, or want to energize yourself.

Ingredients

- 1 beetroot washed, peeled and sliced
- 2 carrots washed and cut
- 2 inch fresh turmeric root peeled
- 1 inch fresh ginger peeled
- 1 tsp lemon juice
- ½ tsp black pepper powder (optional)
- 1 cup almond milk
- 1 cup ice (optional)

Method

Put all ingredients in a blender and blend until smooth

GREEN SMOOTHIE WITH GARLIC, GINGER, AND TURMERIC

A power-packed, extremely healthy smoothie that combines the goodness of greens with medicinal spices that should re-vitalize your brain health.

Ingredients

- ½ inch – 2 inch long fresh cleaned and sliced turmeric root
- ½ inch – 1 inch fresh ginger peeled
- 1 clove garlic
- 1 tsp honey (optional to taste)

- 1 pinch of freshly ground black pepper or pepper powder
- 1 cup of kale
- 1 cup spinach
- 1-2 kiwi peeled
- ½ cup blueberries
- ½ cup sliced cucumber (optional)
- ¼ avocado (optional)
- 3-4 mint leaves
- 1-2 cup filtered water (coconut water may be used as well)
- ½ cup ice

Method

Process all the ingredients in a blender until smooth. Blueberries may be substituted by blackberries depending on your liking. Serves 3-4.

By mixing and matching the "green" ingredients, you may try a couple of different green smoothies. You can substitute cucumber with broccoli.

TROPICAL SMOOTHIE

Basic Ingredients
- 1 banana
- 1 cup pineapple, mango or papaya
- 1 cup Greek yogurt
  ½ cup ice

Optional Ingredients
- 1 tbsp maple syrup

Method

Process all the ingredients in a blender until smooth.

GREEN SMOOTHIE

Basic Ingredients
- 1 cup kale, chopped
- 1 cup spinach
- 1-2 kiwis, peeled
- ½ cup blueberries
- ½ cup Greek yogurt
- ½ cup ice
-

Optional Ingredients
- ½ cup sliced cucumber
- ¼ avocado
- 3-4 mint leaves

Method

Process all the ingredients in a blender until smooth. Blueberries may be substituted with blackberries depending on your liking. Serves 3-4. By mixing and matching the "green" ingredients, you may try a couple of different green smoothies.

VERY BERRY SMOOTHIE

Ingredients
- ½ inch – 1 inch fresh ginger, grated or thinly sliced
- ½ cup blueberries
- ½ cup blackberries
- ½ cup raspberries
- ½ cup strawberries
- 1 cup Greek yogurt
- ½ cup ice

Method

Process all the ingredients in a blender until smooth.

AVOCADO AND GREEK YOGURT DRINK

This is a fusion of Greek and Indian. Mango lassi (mango-yogurt drink) is popular in India. This recipe uses avocado instead of mango and Greek yogurt instead of plain yogurt.

Ingredients
- 1 avocado, pitted, peeled and sliced
- 1 cup Greek yogurt
- ½ cup ice
- 1-2 tablespoon brown sugar or to taste
- 2 cardamom pods (optional)

Method
Process all the ingredients in a blender until smooth.

BRAIN HEALTHY BROTH IDEAS

SPICY VEGAN BROTH

This is a spicy version of the vegan broth that immediately precedes it. It helps with congestion, cold, flu, sore throat, and other ailments due to infections. Like the non-spicy version, this broth also is healing and easy on your gut. The antioxidants and anti-inflammatory compounds in turmeric and ginger make this broth even more healthful.
Ingredients – veggies
- 2-3 celery sticks, cut into inch pieces
- 3 medium tomatoes, chopped
- 1 bell green pepper, cut into pieces
- 1 red bell pepper, cut into pieces
- ¼ of a medium red cabbage, chopped

- 1 large onion, peeled and cut into 1 inch cubes
- ½ cup chopped onion (for sautéing)
- 1 pound (2-3 medium) carrots, washed and cut into pieces
- 1 cup kale
- 1 medium beetroot, washed and cut into pieces

Ingredients – spices and herbs

- ½ cup parsley, chopped
- ½ cup cilantro, chopped
- 3-4 garlic cloves, crushed
- 3-4 whole cloves
- 5-6 black peppercorns or ½ tsp pepper powder
- 1-2 bay leaves
- 1 inch ginger, finely chopped
- 2 tsp turmeric powder or 2 inches of fresh root
- 2 jalapeño peppers, sliced lengthwise (seed in or out depending on your heat tolerance)
- ½ tsp cayenne powder
- ½ tsp cumin powder

Ingredients – other

- 1 gallon water
- Salt to taste (if you must or avoid salt)
- 1 tsp coconut or vegetable oil

Method
1. In a medium pan, heat oil and add onion for sautéing, crushed garlic, ginger, and jalapeño peppers.

2. Sauté for 2-3 minutes or until the onion becomes translucent. Add all the remaining spices (cayenne,

cumin, turmeric, cloves, bay leaves, pepper powder, etc.) and sauté for another 2-3 minutes so the spices are blended well (make sure not to burn them).

3. Transfer the spice mix into a large pot (add some water to wash out any remaining spice mix from the pan and pour it into the large pot.)

4. Add all the vegetables into the pot and add water; bring to a boil.

5. Lower the heat; simmer covered for about 1 hour. Stir occasionally.

6. Once the vegetables are cooked, strain the broth into a large bowl.

7. Add salt to taste, add some chopped fresh herbs of your choice, and serve warm.

8. Refrigerate any remaining broth.

The strained-out vegetables are also nutritious and may be consumed separately.

BONE BROTHS

Bone broth is considered a new age miracle drink. It is gaining popularity with athletes and celebrities as a wellness drink. By combining the immense benefits of nutrients and minerals in traditional bone broth with the medicinal properties of spices and herbs, we can make an even more potent and healthful drink. As explained in Chapter 4 on brain foods (Brain Food #16), there are numerous benefits for bone broth including anti-aging and brain health. When combined with healthful vegetables and medicinal spices and herbs, bone broth indeed becomes a miracle drink that improves your health, boosts immunity, fights diseases and keeps you feeling young.

This is one of the easiest ways to make bone broth. I make it out of the carcass from the rotisserie chicken bought from the departmental store. I remove all the meat and use it as a regular meal for the family and use the entire carcass (without the skins – but skins may be used as well if you prefer) for the bone broth. Not only is this method much simpler but also takes less time, as the chicken bones are already cooked.

Ingredients
- Chicken carcass from a full rotisserie chicken – skin and fat optional
- 4 celery sticks, cut into 1 inch pieces
- 3 medium tomatoes, chopped
- 1 bell pepper, cut into pieces (any color)
- 1 large onion, peeled and quartered
- 1 pound (2-3 medium) carrots, washed and cut into pieces
- ½ cup parsley, chopped
- ½ cup cilantro, chopped
- 3-4 garlic cloves, crushed
- 3-4 whole cloves
- 2 inches ginger, peeled and grated
- 5-6 black peppercorns or ½ tsp pepper powder
- 1-2 bay leaves
- 1 gallon water
- Salt to taste (if you must or avoid salt)

Optional Ingredients
- 2-3 Jalapeño peppers split lengthwise

Method
1. Add everything to a large pot. Bring to a boil
2. Lower the heat; simmer covered for about 2-3 hours.
3. Once the vegetables are fully cooked, strain the broth into a large bowl using a mesh strainer.
4. Add salt to taste, add some chopped fresh herbs of your choice, and serve warm.
5. Refrigerate any remaining broth.

Recipe Notes:

1. The strained vegetables are pretty good and can be eaten after removing all the bone pieces.
2. A slow cooker or pressure cooker may be used for cooking. A pressure cooker will reduce the cooking time if you are in a hurry.
3. You can make this broth a meal by making it a soup. For making it a soup – add ½ cup split lentils and ½ cup brown or white rice to the pot. Add some of the vegetables back and enjoy it when you are recovering from illness and you don't feel like having a full meal. It is very filling and nutritious. This is also a good meal when you are working on a weight loss program.
4. If you like to make this broth spicier, add 1 teaspoon turmeric powder, 1 teaspoon cayenne powder, 1 teaspoon cumin powder and 1 teaspoon fenugreek powder and sauté them in 2 tablespoons of coconut

or olive oil along with onions, garlic, and ginger and add them to the pot where the bones cooked.

5. If you are using fresh bones of any kind, increase the cooking time to 8-24 hours either in a simmering pot or in an instant pot.

6. Optionally, you can add ¼ cup raw unfiltered apple cider vinegar. Apple cider vinegar is known to extract the nutrients from bone into the broth

7. You also make this broth by first roasting fresh bones in an oven at 450 degrees for 45 minutes. Follow the rest of the steps as before.

CHAPTER 6. BRAIN BOOSTING ASIAN RECIPE IDEAS

Asian cuisine, like the Mediterranean and DASH diet focus more on fresh ingredients (as opposed to packaged) and also incorporates spices and herbs known to possess antioxidant, anti-inflammatory, and other benefits. This author's research (explained in the book "Preventing Alzheimer's") found that Asian countries have one of the lowest incidents of Alzheimer's. This author attributes that to healthy foods habits and stronger social connections.

SPINACH/RED CHARD STIR FRY

Basic Ingredients
- 4 cup chopped spinach or red chard
- ½ cup chopped onions
- 4-5 cloves crushed garlic
- 1 tsp turmeric powder
- 2 tsp coconut oil (or vegetable oil)
- Salt to taste
- 1 cup grated coconut

Optional Ingredients
- 2-3 dry red chilies
- 1 spring curry leaves
- ½ tsp mustard seeds
- 1 tsp cumin seeds

Method
1. Heat oil in a nonstick pan. Add optional mustard and cumin seeds and let it splutter.

2. Add onions, garlic, and optional curry leaves and red chilies and sauté for a couple of minutes until onions become translucent.
3. Add turmeric powder and sauté for a couple of minutes more.
4. Now add the chopped spinach or red chard and mix well. Cover and cook for 5-7 minutes, stirring occasionally to make sure no water remains.
5. Add grated coconut and salt, and mix.
6. Cook on low flame for 5 more minutes, stirring occasionally. Switch off the heat once spinach/chard is cooked and no water remains.

Serve as a side dish.

SALMON WITH GREEN MANGO

Basic Ingredients
- 2 lb. skinless salmon, cleaned and cut in 2 inch pieces
- 1-4 tsp chili powder (depending on your tolerance level)
- 1 tsp turmeric
- 1 tsp coriander powder
- ¼ tsp fenugreek powder or ½ tsp fenugreek seeds
- ¼ tsp black pepper powder
- ½ tsp mustard seeds
- 1 medium onion
- 2 tsp ginger root, grated
- 4-5 cloves garlic, crushed
- 2 cups washed and cut green mango (with skin or skin removed depending on your preference)
- 2 cups water (or as required)
- Salt to taste

Optional Ingredients

- 2 sprigs curry leaves
- 2-4 sliced green chilies or jalapeños, seeds removed

Method

1. To make masala paste, combine all the spice powders – chili, turmeric, coriander, fenugreek, and pepper powder – together in a bowl. Add 2 tsp or just enough water to make a thick paste and set aside.
2. Heat oil in a pan and splutter mustard seeds and fenugreek (if seeds are used instead of powder).
3. Add ginger, garlic, onion, and optional green chilies and curry leaves. Sauté until onion becomes translucent.
4. Add the masala paste and mix well on low flame. (Wet the masala to make sure it gets fried but not burnt.)
5. After a few minutes (once masala gets fried), add about 2 cups of water, mix and then add the cut mango pieces.
6. Cover it and bring it to a boil on medium heat. Now add individual fish pieces into the pan.
7. Mix gently, making sure the fish pieces are not broken up and that all the pieces are coated with the gravy.
8. Cover the pan and cook it for about 20 minutes or until fish is done and the gravy is thick. Switch off the flame and keep it covered for 30 minutes for the fish to soak in the spices and mango flavor.

Serve with rice or bread.

Recipe Notes:
1. Paprika may be used instead of chili powder if you desire to make it less spicy.
2. Any other fish may be used instead of salmon.
3. Instead of mango, tamarind or *Garcinia cambogia* (the scientific name for black tamarind available in Asian stores) may be used.
4. Green chilies or jalapeños add more heat to the fish curry. Use it depending on your taste.

BROCCOLI STIR FRY

Basic Ingredients
- 2 lb. broccoli florets washed
- 2 tsp coconut oil (olive oil or vegetable oil can be used instead)
- 1 tsp turmeric powder
- 1 medium onion, sliced
- ¼ tsp black pepper powder
- Salt to taste

Optional Ingredients
- 1 Jalapeño pepper, sliced into thin pieces (seeds out)
- 1 tsp mustard seeds
- ½ cup cilantro
- ½ cup parsley
- ½ tsp fresh lemon juice

Method
1. Heat oil in a medium nonstick pan; crackle optional mustard seeds in oil.

2. Add onion and optional jalapeño pepper. Stir until golden.
3. Add turmeric and black pepper, stir for one minute and then add broccoli florets and mix well until the broccoli is coated with the turmeric.
4. Cover the pan with a lid and cook for 5-10 minutes on low-medium heat stirring occasionally. Once cooked, switch off heat; add the optional cilantro, and parsley. Add salt to taste. Add optional lemon juice.

Mix well and serve hot. Usually, there is no need to add water. At low heat, the moisture in the broccoli will help it to cook well.

COCONUT CURRY CHICKEN

Basic Ingredients

- 1-1/2 pounds chicken breast, cut into small (1 inch) pieces
- 2-4 teaspoons curry powder, depending on your tolerance to the spice
- 1 tsp turmeric
- 1 medium onion, chopped
- 2-3 tsp coconut oil (olive oil or vegetable oil can be used instead)
- ½ tsp pepper powder
- 2 medium potatoes, peeled and cut into 1 inch cubes
- 3-4 cloves garlic, crushed
- ½ inch cube ginger root, peeled and sliced
- 1 can (14 oz.) coconut milk
- ¼ cup mint leaves or cilantro

- Salt to taste
- ½ -1 can chicken broth (depending on the amount of gravy desired)

Optional Ingredients
- 1 cup carrots, sliced
- 2 medium tomatoes, chopped

Method
1. Sprinkle 1 tsp curry powder, ½ tsp turmeric, and ¼ tsp salt on cut chicken. Mix well and set it aside for 10 minutes.
2. In a separate pan, heat oil, sauté onion, garlic, and ginger until onion becomes translucent.
3. Add remaining curry powder, turmeric, and pepper powder. Mix for 1-2 minutes.
4. Add chicken, potatoes, and optional tomatoes and carrots. Mix well 1-2 minutes until the chicken and potatoes are coated with the gravy.
5. Add chicken broth and bring it to a boil. Stir well.
6. Reduce heat to low medium, cover the pan and cook for 10-12 minutes or until chicken, potatoes and carrots are well mixed, the chicken loses its pink color, and potatoes and carrots are about half cooked.
7. Add coconut milk and cover. Simmer on low heat for another 20 minutes or until chicken, potatoes and carrots are cooked well and soft.
8. Add mint leaves/cilantro and stir. Add salt to taste. Switch off the heat and keep it covered for 1-2 minutes before serving.

Serve with rice or bread.

KALE AND CHICKEN FRY

This is something I tried recently and found good. The simplest way to make this is to make chicken with spices following any one of the recipes above, make kale chips and just crumble the chips into the chicken and mix well.
Ingredients

- 2 lbs. boneless chicken breast/beef, cut into 1 inch cubes/strips
- 2 tsp coconut oil (olive oil or vegetable oil can be used instead)
- ½ tsp turmeric powder
- 1-2 tsp black pepper powder
- 2 tsp coriander powder
- 2 large onions, sliced
- 2 inch piece ginger root, thinly sliced
- Salt to taste
- 2-3 medium tomatoes, sliced
- 4-6 cloves garlic, crushed
- 2 cups green or red kale, washed and cut/tore into 1-2 inch pieces (to make kale chips)

Optional Ingredients

- 1 cup cilantro

Method

1. Heat oil in a medium nonstick pan; add onions, garlic, and ginger. Stir until golden.
2. Add coriander powder, pepper powder, and turmeric, stir for one minute, and then add tomatoes and mix well.
3. Add chicken and mix so that chicken is coated well with spices and onions.

4. Cover and simmer for 20-25 minutes or until the chicken is cooked, stirring occasionally so the chicken or the gravy does not stick to the pan.
5. Meanwhile, at the same time, spread the kale pieces on a cookie sheet and put in the oven at 350 degrees for 10 minutes or until the kale pieces become chips and can easily crumble.
6. Once the chicken is cooked, take the kale chips and crumble using your hand and spread on top of the chicken fry.
7. Mix well and cover it for 1 minute. Garnish with cilantro. Serve with rice or naan (Indian bread).

CHAPTER 7: BRAIN BOOSTING SUPPLEMENTS

While most foods described in this book may be used in cooking, some of the brain healthy foods are best taken as supplements. Supplements are available to buy in many online stores such as Amazon and other specialty and nutritional stores. Below are some of the brain-boosting supplements, their typical dosage and popular brands (as per this author):

Turmeric: Turmeric supplements are one of the most popular natural supplements and are usually labeled as "turmeric curcumin" and often includes other ingredients such as black pepper to help absorption and bioavailability. The typical dosage is 1000mg to 1500mg per day. Some turmeric supplements include ginger. Some of the popular brands are Nature Made, Vimerson Health, Bio Shawartz, Physician's CHOICE, NatureWise, and many others.

Garlic: Garlic supplements are widely available and many claims odor control where garlic odor is suppressed. Typical dosage is 1000mg to 2000mg per day. Some of the popular brands are BRI Nutrition, Puritan's Pride, Kyolic, Nature's Bounty and Sundown. Garlic supplement is also available as garlic oil soft gels.

Ginger: Ginger supplements are available as standalone or combined with turmeric. Typical dosage is 1000mg per day. Popular brands are Vimerson Health, Puritan's pride, and Nature's way.

Rosemary: Rosemary supplements are available as rosemary leaves capsules, rosemary extract, and rosemary oil. The typical dosage is 300mg to 600mg.

Sage: Though not as popular as turmeric, ginger or garlic supplements, sage supplements and oil are available to purchase. The typical dosage is 500mg to 1000mg and popular brands are Solaray, Swanson, and Amermed

Ginkgo Biloba: Ginkgo Biloba is available as a stand-alone supplement or paired with other ingredients such as ginseng, bacopa monnieri, and others and promoted as memory and focus enhancing, brain support supplement. There are numerous different brands of Ginkgo Biloba available in the market including Nature's Bounty, NOW, and GreeNatr. The typical dosage is 100mg to 200mg.

Lions Mane: Lions mane supplement is available as capsules, powder or tea bags. Typical dosage is about 2000mg per day. The popular brands for lions mane include Dr Emil Nutrition, Host Defense, The Genius Brand, and Real Mushrooms.

Bacopa Monnieri or Brahmi: Bacopa Monnieri or Brahmi is a popular supplement and is available in capsule form. Typical dosage is 1000mg to 1500mg. The popular brands are Double Wood Supplements, Himalaya Herbal Healthnes and NatureBell among others. Brahmi may also be part of a combined brain boosting formula along with Ginkgo Biloba, Ginseng, and others.

Ashwagandha: Ashwagandha is one of the more popular supplements. The most common brands are Physician's Choice, Nutririse, Nutraherbals, Organic India, and many more. Typical dosage is 500mg – 1000mg per day.

Ginseng: Ginseng is another popular supplement. Many vendors offer ginseng extract in the form of capsules. Some vendors offer ginseng in the dry root form and sliced into pieces. These may be used for making ginseng tea. Typical dosage is 1000mg – 1500mg. Popular brands include NutraChamps, Nature's Bounty, Auragin, Herbtronics, NOW and many others.

Gotu Kola or Indian Pennywort: Gotu Kola is less popular as a stand-alone supplement. However, users who take Gotu Kola swear by its ability in reducing anxiety and improving mental clarity among others. The typical dosage is about 400mg – 800mg per day. The popular brands are Nature's Way, Pure Mountain Botanicals, Organic India among others.

Lemon balm: Lemon balm is a popular supplement and is available as capsules, liquid extract and some cases roll on for blister, bug bites, etc. For improving memory and alertness, capsule formulation is recommended. The typical dosage is 600mg – 1200mg per day. The popular brands include Oregon's Wild, Fresh Nutrition, New Chapter, etc.

Fish Oil: Fish oil supplements are a rich source of Omega-3 fatty acids - Docosahexaenoic acid (DHA) and eicosapentaenoic acid (EPA). DHA plays a very important role in maintaining brain health and function. DHA accounts for a quarter of total fat and about 90% of omega-3 fat found in your brain cells. While EPA does not directly contribute to brain function, it helps with depression, improved mode, and focus. Omega-3 fatty acids also have antioxidant and anti-inflammatory properties which improve overall health and keeps the brain from oxidative damage and inflammation. The typical dosage for fish oil is about 1000mg per day. There are numerous vendors selling fish oil supplements, so it is hard to list popular ones.

Resveratrol: Resveratrol is naturally occurring antioxidant found mainly in colored (purple and red primarily) fruits and vegetables. Some of the sources of resveratrol include red grapes, raspberries, blueberries and eggplants, Resveratrol is also found in red wine, chocolates and nuts like peanuts. Resveratrol is believed to maintain the health of the hippocampus, the part of the brain associated with memory. The typical dosage of resveratrol is 1000mg to 2000mg per day.

Other supplements:
Phosphatidylserine – It is a type of fat compound that if found in the brain and is considered to be helpful in maintaining brain health. Typical dosage 200mg-400mg
Acetyl-L-Carnitine: It is an amino acid and helps with metabolism and energy production resulting in improved focus and slow down memory loss. Typical dosage 1000mg-2000mg.
Creatine – Creatine is found in meat, fish, and eggs and can improve memory and thought process. Typical dosage about 1500mg-3000mg.
Rhodiola Rosea – It is derived from the Chinese herb of the same name. It can reduce fatigue and improve brain function. Typical dosage 300mg-500mg

While many of the above supplements are available as capsules, some are available in teabag form or in powder form. You can make tea by steeping these tea bags in hot/boiling water for about 3-6 minutes. If you are getting powder, these powders may be added to smoothies to convert an ordinary smoothie to a brain-boosting one.

Note About Dietary Supplement Market:

The dietary supplement market is not as regulated as the regular drug market. There are also numerous companies offering different supplements with wide-ranging and often wild claims. It is important to stick with trusted brands if you choose to go for supplements. If you are purchasing online, make sure that it is from a trusted brand. My recommendation is to start shopping supplements by going to one of the larger/reputed General nutritional stores first before starting to shop online. If a reputed store is willing to bet their reputation on the supplement, that provides one proof point. Also, you get to talk to someone at the store.

Always, consult a physician if you plan to take supplements long term or you are pregnant or breast-feeding.

Also, note that the brands listed for supplements are some of the known or popular brands at the time writing this book. This may change in the future and the author is no way endorsing any of the brands. Please do your research before buying any dietary supplements.

CHAPTER 8: SUMMARY

I hope this book provides you with some ideas of foods that help in maintaining a healthy brain. A healthy brain a huge part of any anti-aging regimen and also helps or slows down age-related brain disorders such as dementia, Alzheimer's, and Parkinson's. The primary focus in this book is on maintaining a healthy brain through food by improving the blood flow to brain, reducing the likelihood plaque build-up, and reducing the rate of brain shrinkage.

Some of the key points from the various foods and diet plans discussed in this book are summarized below:

1. Eat more of the brain foods identified in this book.
2. Eat more colorful vegetables and fruits (Mediterranean/DASH)
3. Limit/avoid processed foods (DASH Diet/ Mediterranean)
4. Use healthy oils such as olive oil/coconut oil (Mediterranean)
5. Limit/avoid sodas of any kind (common sense diet)
6. Eat more vegan and organic protein.
7. Limit sugar intake (common sense diet)
8. Limit alcohol consumption (common sense diet)
9. Limit salt. Be aware many off the shelf and processed foods have too much sodium (DASH Diet)
10. Eat freshly prepared foods whenever possible. Cook at home more often. It makes not only short term and long-term economic sense but is healthful as well (common sense diet)
11. Use spices and herbs – especially turmeric, garlic and ginger (and others such as cinnamon, chili powder, etc.) – in the preparation of foods that help

fight inflammation and neutralize free radicals
(South Asian)
12. Use herbs that help with cognition and memory
(Asian and Chinese herbs)
13. Go for supplements if you think there are not
enough brain nourishing foods in your regular diet

Brain function, brain capabilities, and memory may further be improved by the proper brain or mental exercises. Here is my list of the top 3 things to keep and active brain/mind and improve brain function

1. Be a lifelong learner, be active mentally

- Learn something new every day, every week, every month. Look back at the end of the day and think about what you learned that day. As part of your New Year's resolutions, plan to learn one new skill a year. It could be:

    a. Learn a musical instrument.

    b. Learn a new language.

    c. Learn a new hobby such as knitting or crocheting.

    d. Learning chess, checkers, or any strategy game.

    e. Learn a new subject or topic related to your work.

- Keep mentally active.

> f. Play games such as sudoku, scrabble, ken-ken, crossword puzzles, or cards.
>
> g. Play brain teasers and trivia games
>
> h. Play games on Lumosity or other brain training apps.
>
> i. Keep a diary or journal to write down daily experiences of "who, what, where, when, and why". The process of writing things down helps to improve memory. Describe everything as vividly as possible. Visualize the events before writing them down.
>
> j. Practice memorization. Take it up as a hobby. Try to remember names, numbers (phone number, credit card number), and facts (state names, country names, capitals). Visualize and associate names with people and objects.

2. **Be physically active.**

- Be aware of how much time you exercise, and how much time you sit on the sofa or sit at the workplace.
- Exercise at least 30 minutes a day. Pick up a physical activity that you enjoy. Enlist other people so you can exercise in groups or teams where you can feed off each other and maintain the motivation.
- Hit the gym or pick up running, walking, or a team game such as tennis, volleyball, basketball, etc.
- Join senior leagues for sports and physical activities.
- Practice yoga or tai chi, which provide many benefits including:

- ○ improved balance and coordination that help in your old age; especially your balance is impacted by Alzheimer's
- ○ stress reduction again, they help in reducing stress on the brain

3. Improve the quality of sleep.

- Sleep time is used by the brain for memory formation. The whole body uses sleep as a restorative process to recover from all the work the body did during the hours awake.

- Sleep helps to flush out toxins from the brain and prevent the formation of beta-amyloid plaques in the brain that increases risk for Alzheimer's.

DISCLAIMER

This book details the author's personal experiences in using Indian spices and information contained in the public domain, as well as the author's opinion. The author is not licensed as a doctor, nutritionist or chef. The author is providing this book and its contents on an "as is" basis and makes no representations or warranties of any kind with respect to this book or its contents. The author disclaims all such representations and warranties, including for example warranties of merchantability and educational or medical advice for a particular purpose. In addition, the author does not represent or warrant that the information accessible via this book is accurate, complete or current. The statements made about products and services have not been evaluated by the US FDA or any equivalent organization in other countries.

The author will not be liable for damages arising out of or in connection with the use of this book or the information contained within. This is a comprehensive limitation of liability that applies to all damages of any kind, including (without limitation) compensatory; direct, indirect or consequential damages; loss of data, income or profit; loss of or damage to property and claims of third parties. It is understood that this book is not intended as a substitute for consultation with a licensed medical or a culinary professional. Before starting any lifestyle changes, it is recommended that you consult a licensed professional to ensure that you are doing what's best for your situation. The use of this book implies your acceptance of this disclaimer.

Thank You

If you enjoyed this book or found it useful, I would greatly appreciate if you could post a short review on Amazon. I read all the reviews and your feedback will help me to make this book even better. For your convenience, please click or type in the following link to take you directly to Amazon where you can post the review:https://www.amazon.com/dp/B07YBQY7JW

APPENDIX I. SOURCES AND REFERENCES

This book was written based on the author's personal experience with super foods and spices as well as information from a wide range of sources. Some of the key sources are outlined below, in case the reader would like to read more details about Alzheimer's and its prevention.

15 Brain Foods That Boost Memory
https://draxe.com/15-brain-foods-to-boost-focus-and-memory/
Health benefits of Eggs
https://www.huffingtonpost.com/2013/03/30/health-benefits-of-eggs-yolks_n_2966554.html

Leafy green vegetables and brain health
https://consumer.healthday.com/senior-citizen-information-31/misc-aging-news-10/lots-of-leafy-greens-might-shield-aging-brains-study-finds-697909.html

Walnuts and memory
https://www.huffingtonpost.com/2015/01/22/walnuts-boost-memory-study_n_6525316.html

6 brain foods good for the mind
http://www.telegraph.co.uk/news/science/science-news/11364896/Brain-food-6-snacks-that-are-good-for-the-mind.html

Eat smart for a healthier brain
https://www.webmd.com/diet/features/eat-smart-healthier-brain#1

Omega-3 fatty acids and their role in central nervous system https://www.ncbi.nlm.nih.gov/pubmed/26795198

Vitamin B12 and Omega-3 effects on brain function
https://www.ncbi.nlm.nih.gov/pubmed/26809263

Fish consumption and cognitive decline with age
https://www.ncbi.nlm.nih.gov/pubmed/16216930

Neuro-protective effects of berries on neurodegenerative diseases
https://www.ncbi.nlm.nih.gov/pmc/articles/PMC4192974/

Blueberries improve memory in older adults
https://www.ncbi.nlm.nih.gov/pmc/articles/PMC2850944/

Neuroprotective properties of turmeric
http://www.eurekaselect.com/76132
http://www.nature.com/articles/srep38846
http://articles.mercola.com/sites/articles/archive/2013/07/08/-vs-drugs-for-parkinsons.aspx
http://www.sciencedirect.com/science/article/pii/S1357272508002550

Anti-inflammatory properties of turmeric
https://www.ncbi.nlm.nih.gov/pubmed/19594223
https://www.ncbi.nlm.nih.gov/pubmed/12676044

Broccoli benefits
https://www.ncbi.nlm.nih.gov/pmc/articles/PMC3725709/

Chocolate intake associated with better cognitive function
https://www.ncbi.nlm.nih.gov/pubmed/26873453

Nuts and cognitive function
https://www.ncbi.nlm.nih.gov/pmc/articles/PMC4105147/

10 foods to boost your brain power
https://www.bbcgoodfood.com/howto/guide/10-foods-boost-your-brainpower

**https://www.merckmanuals.com/home/older-people's-health-issues/the-aging-body/changes-in-the-body-with-aging
https://medlineplus.gov/ency/article/004012.htm**

DASH diet with exercise benefits cognition.

https://www.alzdiscovery.org/cognitive-vitality/blog/exercise-with-dash-diet-improved-cognitive-functions-in-older-adults

https://www.webmd.com/hypertension-high-blood-pressure/news/20100308/dash-diet-fuels-the-brain

PREVIEW OF OTHER BOOKS IN THIS SERIES

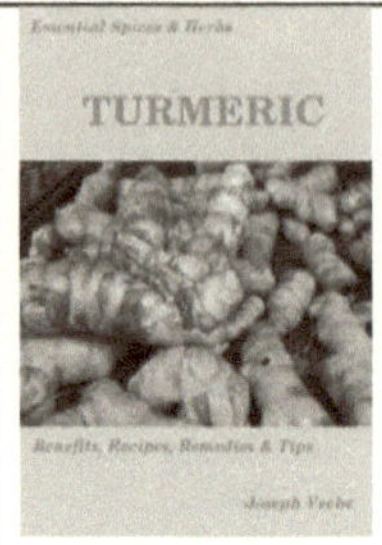	This book Contains: • Many health benefits of turmeric including fighting cancer, inflammation and pain. • Turmeric as beauty treatments - turmeric masks • Recipes for teas, smoothies and dishes • References and links to a number of research studies on the effectiveness of turmeric
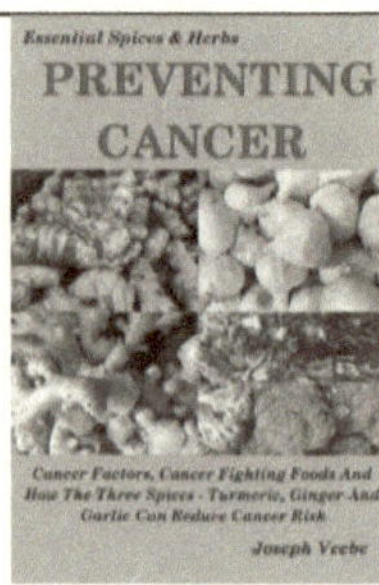	The book includes: • Cancer causing factors and how to avoid them • Top 12 cancer fighting foods, the cancers they fight and how to incorporate them into your diet • Cancer fighting benefits of Turmeric, Ginger and Garlic • Over 30 recipes including teas, smoothies and other dishes that incorporate these spices
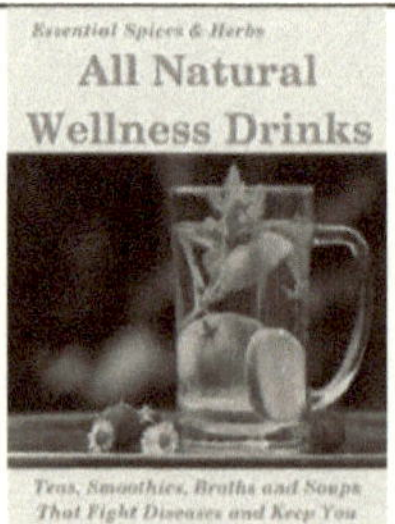	Contains 35 recipes for wellness drinks that includes teas, smoothies, soups and vegan & bone broths. The recipes in this book are unique and combine super foods, medicinal spices and herbs. These drinks are anti-cancer, anti-diabetic, ant-aging, heart healthy, anti-inflammatory and antioxidant as well as promote weight loss.

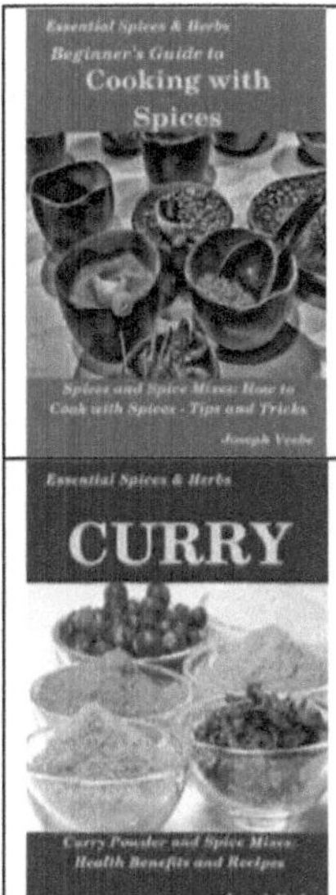	Find out how to start using spices as seasoning and health ingredient. Includes sample recipes. Beginner's guide to cooking with spices is an introductory book that explains the history, various uses and their medicinal properties and health benefits. The book details how they may be easily incorporated in everyday cooking.
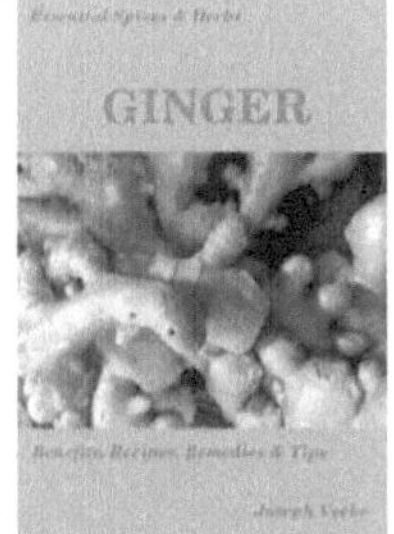	Curry powder contains turmeric, chili powder, coriander and cumin among others.This book includes: • History of curry and curry powder • Health benefits of each ingredients • How to make various curry powder and curry paste mixes including Indian, Thai and Ethiopian curry mixes • Several recipes for making Indian and Thai curries
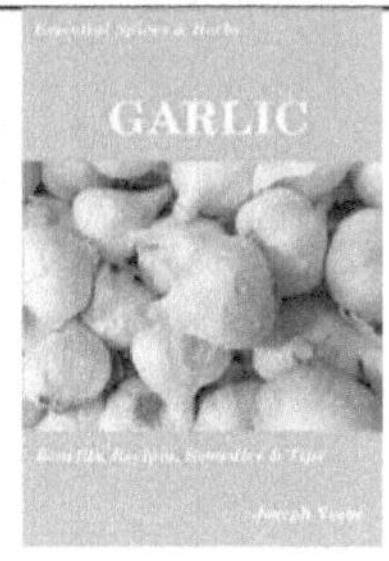	The book details: • Many health benefits of ginger including fighting cancer, inflammation, pain and nausea • Remedies using ginger • Recipes for teas, smoothies and dishes • References and links
	• Many health benefits of garlic including fighting cancer, inflammation, heart health and more • Remedies using garlic • Recipes for teas, smoothies and dishes • References and links

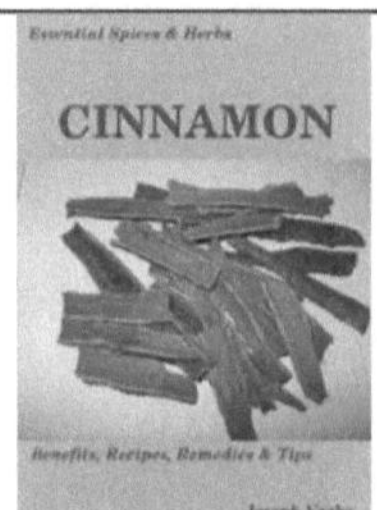	This book contains: • Many health benefits of cinnamon including anti-diabetic, neuroprotective and others • Recipes for teas, smoothies and dishes • References
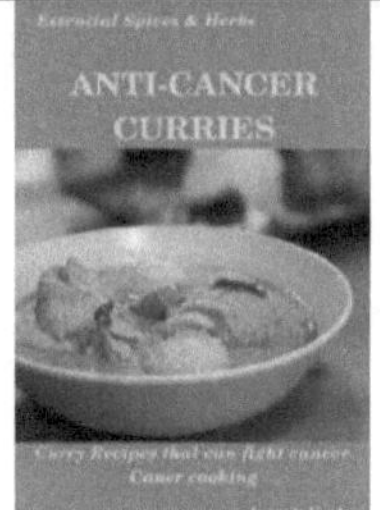	Curry powder contains turmeric, chili powder, coriander and cumin among others. They are all known to have immense health benefits. This book contains 30 curry recipes that uses healthy and anti-cancer ingredients. These recipes are simple and takes an average of 20-30 minutes to prepare.
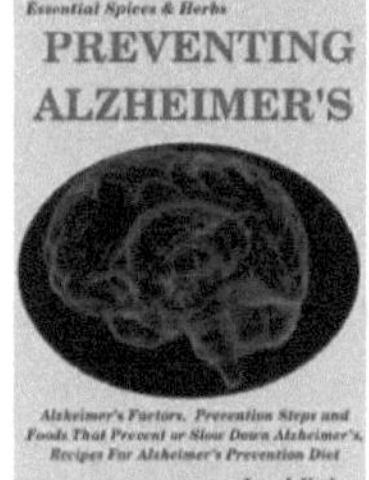	Preventing Alzheimer's offers a quick insight into Alzheimer's causing factors, various steps to reduce risk, and ways to prevent or slow down the progression of the disease. A list of foods that help protect brain and boost brain health and over 30 recipes are included in the book.
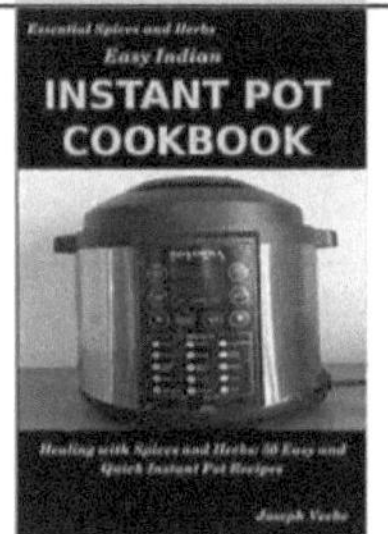	Easy and healthy instant pot recipes for making Indian food. They are simplistic and easy to make and taste as close to authentic Indian food but with much less effort.